100 Questions and Answers About Gender Identity

The Transgender, Nonbinary, Gender-Fluid and Queer Spectrum

Michigan State University School of Journalism

Read The Spirit Books
an imprint of
David Crumm Media, LLC
Canton, Michigan

For more information and further discussion, visit

news.jrn.msu.edu/culturalcompetence/

Cover art and design by
Rick Nease
www.RickNeaseArt.com

Published By
Read The Spirit Books
an imprint of
David Crumm Media, LLC
42015 Ford Rd., Suite 234
Canton, Michigan, USA

For information about customized editions, bulk
purchases or permissions, contact David Crumm
Media, LLC at info@DavidCrummMedia.com

Contents

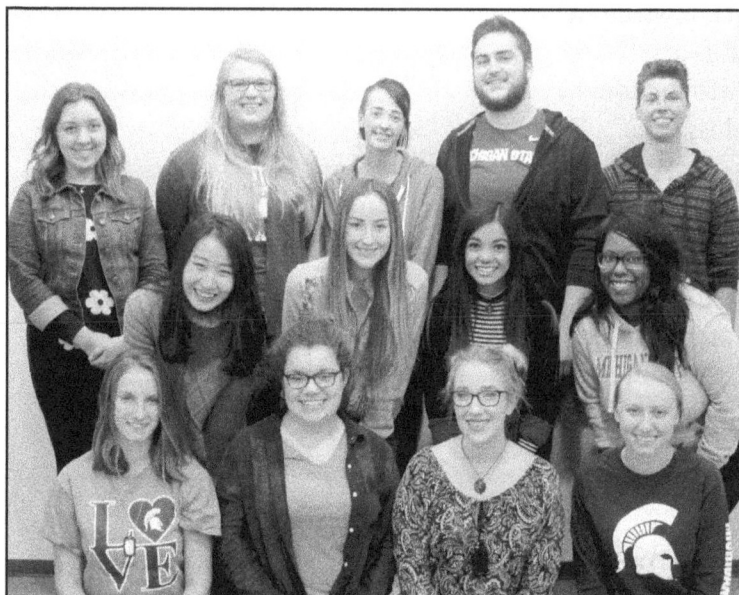

The authors of this guide, front row from left: Mikayla DeMers, Vaughn Rose Springer, Rene Kiss and Alexis Stark. Middle row: Bingqing Mao, Jessica Pack, Terri Powys and Paige Boyd. Back row: Savannah Swix, Rebecca Isabelle Fadler, Caitlin Taylor, Christopher Boggus and Kalib Watson.

Acknowledgments

Many organizations and individuals helped make this guide. Our first ally was Michigan State University's Lesbian, Bisexual, Gay, and Transgender Resource Center. Thanks to Director Deanna "Dee" Hurlbert, who suggested this guide. Assistant Director Alex C. Lange helped every step of the way providing early guidance, meeting with us in the classroom and critiquing drafts. Months before the class began, the National Center for Transgender Equality's media relations manager, Jay Wu, advised us. They told us that a big study was being analyzed. In a wonderful coincidence, on our last day of class the center released the largest survey ever on transgender people. With that data, we updated this guide in many places to reflect the online survey's findings from 27,715 adults. More than 300 transgender, LBGTQ+ and allied organizations helped circulate the survey or word about it. About a third of respondents identified as nonbinary. The U.S. Transgender Survey report makes many comparisons of transgender people's perspectives with those of the overall U.S. population and we recommend it highly. The report is at http://www.ustranssurvey.org/report.

Our first guest speaker was Nathan Triplett, director of public policy and political action for Equality Michigan. For our last class, PFLAG Detroit spokeswoman Rachael Jackson drove through snow to help us.

When we asked Bré Anne Campbell, co-founder and executive director of the Trans Sistas of Color Project – Detroit, for a guest speaker, she brought a panel. It included Jeynce Poindexter, Cierra Burks, Alexandria Gibson, Tamisha Rembert and Latrice Ward. An audience of 125 students and faculty members came to hear them. Some of their questions are in this guide.

The covers feature several of our advisers. On the front cover, from left, are Alex Lange (photo by Hannah Brenner), Hunter Keith and his mother, Roz Gould Keith, and Rachael Jackson (photo by Jeremy Steele). Keith, founder and president of Stand with Trans, was also one of our readers. Alexandria Gibson and Tamisha Rembert are on the back cover.

Stephanie Nawyn, co-director for MSU's Center for Gender in Global Context, helped with the Trans Sistas event and the resources section. Nawyn is also co-director for Academic Programs, Outreach and Engagement at MSU.

MSU's Kristen A. Renn, professor of Higher, Adult, and Lifelong Education in the Department of Educational Administration, also advised. She is associate dean of Undergraduate Studies and director for Student Success Initiatives.

Others who helped were Rosie Priest of PFLAG Detroit and Michelle Fox-Phillips, a co-founder of both

Transgender Michigan and Transgender Detroit. Diane Schultz, secretary of Detroit's Gender-Identity Alliance Network, also supported us. We thank the people at Affirmations in Ferndale, Michigan.

Amy Hunter, transgender advocacy project coordinator for ACLU Michigan, pointed us to great people and resources.

Dr. Christy Duan, general adult psychiatry intern at Northwell Health in Great Neck, New York, was an early supporter and a reader on the project.

Bethany Grace Howe, University of Oregon educator and journalist, also critiqued the content. Adam Pawlus, executive director of the National Lesbian and Gay Journalists Association, referred us to Howe.

Richard Epps, Michigan State University School of Journalism web and publication design professor, directed graphics production. Professor Darcy Greene helped with photography.

Finally, we thank School of Journalism Director and Professor Lucinda Davenport, who has supported this series from the beginning.

Preface

Chances are that you've met a transgender person, even if you didn't know it.

Transgender people have been around forever, and we come from all walks of life, work in a wide range of occupations, and are parts of all kinds of communities. According to our best estimates, there are nearly 2 million transgender people living, working and going to school all over the United States.

For many Americans, it might seem like transgender people are a new phenomenon, because we and the issues we face in society have taken center stage in politics, pop culture, and the press only in the last few years. As more and more people become familiar with who transgender people are—whether through following advocacy for non-discrimination laws or celebrity news—acceptance of transgender people increases as well. Unfortunately, this has also led to backlash in the form of anti-transgender political initiatives, including "bathroom ban" legislation and President Donald Trump's ban on transgender people serving openly in the military.

The media has been and continues to be a crucial means for people to learn about who transgender people are and to gain an understanding of the transgender community's most urgent needs. In order to report fairly on transgender people without sensationalizing or misrepresenting us, however, reporters must have a good grounding in these issues too. This guide is an important resource for journalists who are looking to lay that foundation to ensure that their reporting on transgender issues is as accurate and balanced as possible. After all, reporters are among those who must deal with the thorniest of situations, such as responding to the tragic epidemic of lethal violence against transgender people, particularly transgender women of color.

Transgender people will only become a larger part of the public conversation as time goes on, and it is crucial that we are well-represented in that conversation.

Mara Keisling
Executive Director,
National Center for
Transgender
Equality
September 2017

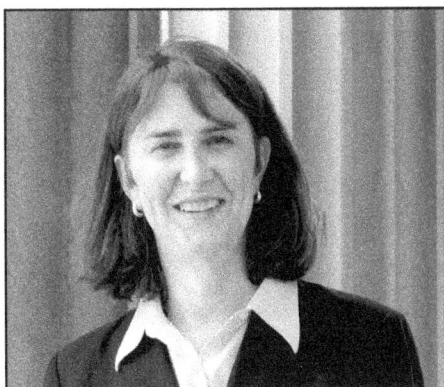

Introduction

We live in a time of rapid change for gender identity rights. Change is happening so quickly and visibility is increasing so rapidly it can be difficult to keep up. People of marginalized gender identities seek to live authentically and have asked for greater visibility and respect. Legislation is rewriting U.S. law books. Language and labels, always fluid, are evolving quickly. New terms, even pronouns, are developing to fill the vacuum about how to refer to people.

The statement that "The T is no longer silent," has two meanings. One is that transgender people want to be visible and accepted. Another is a desire for full involvement in the LGBTQ+ movement for recognition and rights.

Sexual orientation and gender identity are not the same. Another guide in this series, "100 Questions and Answers About Sexual Orientation," covers sexuality. People represented in both guides have shared aspirations.

One reason for growing acceptance of gay rights has been personal relationships. For several reasons, however, transgender people are still less visible than some other LGBTQ+ groups. In 2016, the Pew Research Center found that 87 percent of people surveyed said they knew someone who is gay or lesbian. Only about a third as many said they knew someone who is transgender.

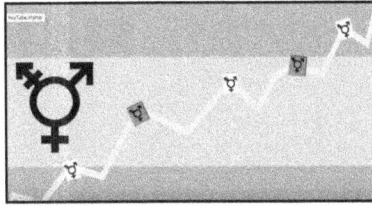

View the Bias Busters video at: http://bit.ly/2iEA5Oq **or scan the code below**

While recognition of LBGTQ+ rights is changing quickly, it did not start yesterday. It has been building for decades.

With change, people seek answers by asking questions. Students in a Michigan State University journalism class gathered these questions from interviews with transgender people, nonbinary people and others. The students then researched the answers. The guide was helped tremendously by the U.S. Transgender Survey, which we cite frequently. Finally, expert allies checked the work for accuracy.

Our goal is to help people find accurate, authoritative and respectful answers to their basic questions. With these answers and resources, we hope to encourage conversations that are not harmful or uncomfortable.

We encourage you to have those conversations and hope this guide can be a small step in your journey.

Joe Grimm
Series editor
School of Journalism
Michigan State University

Glossary

Gender-identity language is one of the most rapidly changing parts of the English language. Language around gender identity is still evolving and has not been codified. This means some of these terms may become less preferred or obsolete within a few years. This glossary is meant to help you in this book and with conversations.

agender A person who identifies as neither male nor female. Not the same as asexual.

androgynous To have both feminine and masculine characteristics.

asexual Having no apparent sex or sex organs, or having no interest in sexual activity.

bigender Having two or more gender identities at the same time, or that fluctuate.

Chicanx (chi-CAHN-ex) A gender-neutral substitute for the feminine Chicana and masculine Chicano.

cisgender When one's gender aligns with their sex as assigned at birth. The Latin prefix cis means "on the same side of." It is the inverse of trans and gives us a word that is needed in some conversations.

crossdresser A person who sometimes wears clothes, accessories and makeup associated with a different gender. These are usually heterosexual cisgender males. This is a form of gender expression and is not done to entertain others.

drag queen or king A man who dresses as a woman, or a woman who dresses as a man to entertain at a club or show.

gender-confirmation surgery Helps people physically align their body with their gender identity. Surgery is not a requirement of being transgender. Gender-reassignment surgery is another term that is sometimes used, but is falling out of favor.

gender dysphoria Emotional or mental distress one feels when gender identity does not match the sex assigned at birth. Gender dysphoria replaced the clinical diagnosis of "gender identity disorder" in 2012. It is defined as "longstanding discomfort with the incongruence between gender identity and external sexual anatomy at birth along with interference with social, school, or other areas of function." Not all transgender people have gender dysphoria.

gender expression How people present their gender to others. This can include clothing, grooming and how they act.

gender fluid A gender identity that changes over time. Someone who is gender fluid may variously identify as a man, woman, non-binary, or a combination.

gender identity People's knowledge of who they are -- man, woman, both, neither -- and how they call themselves.

gender-neutral pronouns These identify people as neither male nor female and can include those who identify as a combination or neither. These pronouns are used most often but are not the only ones being tried:

    they/them/theirs (used as singulars)
    ve/vir/virs
    ze/zir/zirs

Because we cannot assume gender identity on sight, it is better not to assume and to ask or to listen during introductions.

gender-nonconforming People who do not look or act in the ways stereotypically expected of their birth-assigned sex. Also called gender expansive.

genderqueer People who do not identify exclusively with male or female characteristics. Their gender might be neither male nor female.

intersex Having anatomical characteristics traditionally associated with both sexes. Hermaphrodite is a dated term for this and can offend.

Latinx (lah-TEEN-ex) A gender-neutral substitute for the feminine Latina and masculine Latino.

Mx. (meks or miks) A gender-neutral alternative to Mr., Ms. and Miss.

nonbinary Describes people who do not identify as exclusively only male or female.

outing Disclosing that someone is transgender when they have not disclosed it themselves.

passing A transgender person who is perceived as cisgender.

transgender One whose gender is different from their sex assigned at birth. It is an adjective and can offend if used as a noun. While this guide usually uses transgender for consistency, trans is also accepted.

transgender female/feminine/woman A person whose birth sex is male, but who identifies as a woman. Sometimes referred to as MTF (male to female), though this usage is dated. Newer terms are AMAB (assigned male at birth), MAAB (male assigned at birth) or DMAB (designated male at birth).

transgender male/masculine/man A person whose birth sex is female, but who identifies as a man. Sometimes referred to as FTM (female to male), a dated usage. Newer terms are AFAB (assigned female at birth), FAAB (female assigned at birth) or DFAB (designated female at birth).

transition The process of changing from the gender identity congruent with the sex assigned at birth to another gender identity. The process can be long, and there are many ways to transition. It can include changing names and documents, how one presents oneself in public and different medical procedures.

transsexual Some consider this to be an outdated term for transgender.

two-spirit Mostly used by indigenous cultures, this refers to a person who possesses male and female identities.

Gender and Sex

1 What is the difference between gender and sex?

Sex is assigned at birth, primarily on the basis of external anatomy. Possible labels are male, female or intersex. Gender is one's internal knowledge of who they are, whether that be man, woman, transgender, genderfluid, nonbinary or another term.

2 What is the gender spectrum?

The Trevor Project states that gender is fluid and can change depending on how people perceive themselves. The gender identity spectrum illustrates that gender has many dimensions. The gender spectrum is someone's knowledge of their gender. The expression spectrum shows how people present their gender. The presentation spectrum shows how the world perceives them. Transgender, nonbinary and cisgender identities can be anywhere along the spectrum or even beyond it.

The Spectrum

BIOLOGICAL SEX
(What the doctor assigns you at birth)

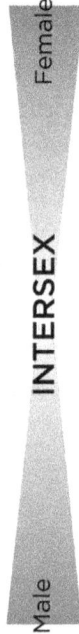

Male — Intersex — Female

SEXUAL ORIENTATION
(Who you like)

Attracted to women — BISEXUAL ASEXUAL PANSEXUAL — Attracted to men

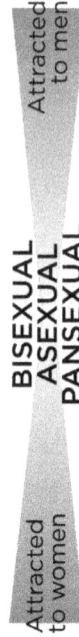

GENDER IDENTITY
(How you feel on the inside)

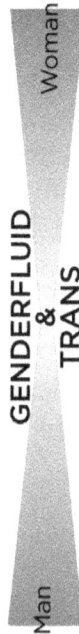

Man — GENDERFLUID & TRANS — Woman

GENDER EXPRESSION
(How you present yourself to others)

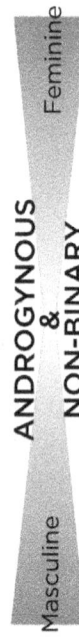

Masculine — ANDROGYNOUS & NON-BINARY — Feminine

GENDER PRESENTATION
(How the world sees you)

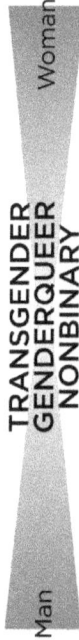

Man — TRANSGENDER GENDERQUEER NONBINARY — Woman

3 At what age do people start understanding their own gender identity?

The U.S. Transgender Survey reported that 32 percent of respondents said they began by age 5 to feel that their assigned sex did not match their gender identity. An additional 28 percent, for a total of 60 percent, began to feel that way by age 10. Acting outside of typical gender roles is called gender-nonconforming behavior. Children who exhibit this may not be transgender, but it can be a sign. A better guideline is if the child is consistent, insistent and persistent about their identity. Then they might be transgender.

4 What is transitioning?

This is the process of moving from the sex assigned at birth with all that it implies to a gender consistent with someone's identity. The elements of transitioning vary. Some people begin transitioning with a new name or pronouns. Others might change their hairstyle, change the way they dress, or start or stop wearing makeup. Some arrange for hormone therapy or surgery.

5 How does someone know they should transition?

According to the National Center for Transgender Equality, awareness can come at any age. It usually

Procedures in the Transgender Community

Respondents were asked a series of questions about whether they received or wanted specific surgical and other procedures. Respondents received different questions based on the sex that they reported was listed on their original birth certificate.

...among Transgender Men

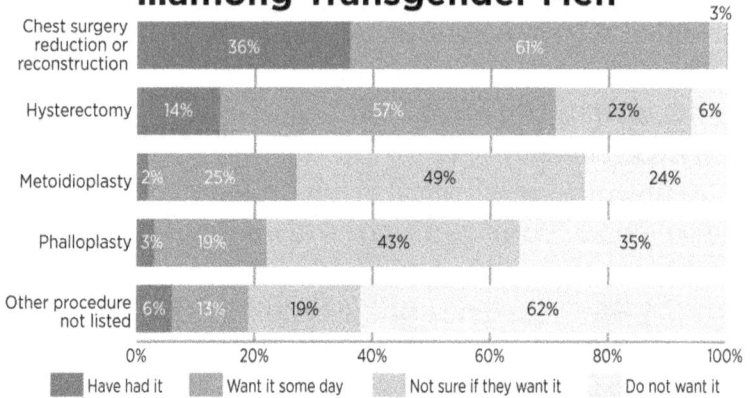

Procedure	Have had it	Want it some day	Not sure if they want it	Do not want it
Chest surgery reduction or reconstruction	36%	61%		3%
Hysterectomy	14%	57%	23%	6%
Metoidioplasty	2%	25%	49%	24%
Phalloplasty	3%	19%	43%	35%
Other procedure not listed	6%	13%	19%	62%

0%   20%   40%   60%   80%   100%

■ Have had it   ■ Want it some day   ■ Not sure if they want it   ■ Do not want it

...among Transgender Women

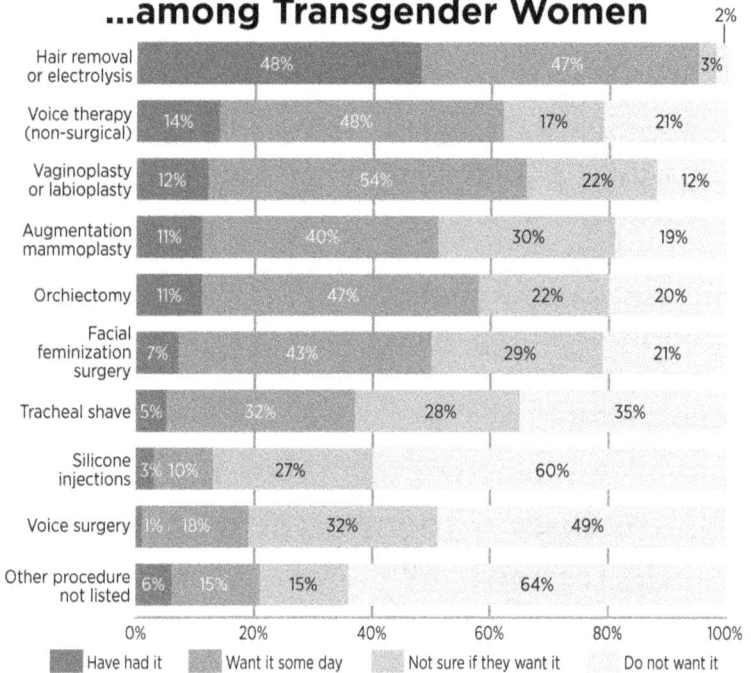

Procedure	Have had it	Want it some day	Not sure if they want it	Do not want it
Hair removal or electrolysis	48%	47%		2% / 3%
Voice therapy (non-surgical)	14%	48%	17%	21%
Vaginoplasty or labioplasty	12%	54%	22%	12%
Augmentation mammoplasty	11%	40%	30%	19%
Orchiectomy	11%	47%	22%	20%
Facial feminization surgery	7%	43%	29%	21%
Tracheal shave	5%	32%	28%	35%
Silicone injections	3%	10%	27%	60%
Voice surgery	1%	18%	32%	49%
Other procedure not listed	6%	15%	15%	64%

0%   20%   40%   60%   80%   100%

■ Have had it   ■ Want it some day   ■ Not sure if they want it   ■ Do not want it

Source US Transgender Survey   Graphic by Rachel Beard

starts with a struggle to understand. This can include reflection, confusion and denial. Transitioning comes at a cost, so it is not an easy decision to make. It can mean the loss of important relationships. It can also lead to stigma and physical or verbal harassment. Some people never openly transition. Others do in hopes of ending the confusion and being more open and honest with themselves and others.

6 Do all transgender people have gender-confirming surgery?

Most do not. According to the U.S. Transgender Survey, only 25 percent of respondents said they had some type of gender-confirming surgery. Transgender men were more likely than transgender women to have had surgery, 42 percent to 28 percent. Nine percent of nonbinary people have had surgery. Fourteen percent of transgender women and 21 percent of transgender men said they never wanted surgery. Surgery is expensive and insurance doesn't always cover it. Even if a transgender person does not have or want surgery, their identity is still valid.

7 Are most transgender people gay?

This question is about the intersection of gender identity and sexual attraction. First, changing gender does not change other characteristics about a person. That includes whom they are attracted to. Also, not all people experience sexual attraction and not all are attracted to just one sex.

Identity

8 What is gender identity?

Gender identity is an individual's knowledge of who they are and how they identify themselves. It is deeply engrained in their sense of self. A person can identify as a woman, a man, nonbinary, gender-fluid or as having no gender. Gender is not based on physical characteristics, chromosomes, hormones or sexuality.

9 How many transgender people are there in the United States?

This number is affected by how safe and comfortable people feel in reporting that they are transgender. According to a UCLA Williams Institute analysis of federal and state data, an estimated 1.4 million U.S. adults identify as transgender. That is about 0.6 percent of the adult population. It does not include youth. Some gender-nonconforming or nonbinary people identify themselves as trans. Others just don't disclose their gender identities.

10 How racially diverse is the transgender population?

In 2016, UCLA's Williams Institute found that the transgender population is more racially and ethnically diverse than the U.S. general population. It reported that 55 percent of adults who said they were transgender identified as White, 21 percent identified as Latino or Hispanic, 16 percent identified as African American or Black and 8 percent identified as another race or ethnicity. In every racial group, fewer than 1 percent said they were transgender.

11 What is "deadnaming?"

"Deadnaming" is referring to a transgender person by their birth name instead of their new name. It can be out of habit or by accident or it can signal rejection of the person's identity. Even asking a person about their "birth name" or "old name" can hurt. Questioning identity in such a personal way can resurface gender dysphoria, or negative experiences associated with their transition. It is respectful to address all people by the name they prefer.

12 What issues do transgender people have with body image?

All people, regardless of gender identity, can experience insecurities about their bodies. Insecurities can be about weight, facial features and presence or absence of body parts or genitalia. Such issues can be magnified for transgender people trying to fit social standards of masculinity and femininity.

13 Which happens more, male to female or female to male?

Because gender is not strictly binary, some people fit neither category. People can be nonbinary or gender-fluid and might be neither entirely male or female. New research asks people about their sex assigned at birth and how they identify now, but descriptions of gender identity are becoming more detailed and fluid. Various studies have shown male-to-female transitions occur two to four times more frequently than female-to-male transitions. The U.S. Transgender Survey was not designed to estimate proportions. Its respondents were 29 percent transgender men, 33 percent transgender women, 35 percent nonbinary and 3 percent crossdresssers.

14 How often do intersex births occur?

The Intersex Society of North America says the exact number is not known because the definition of intersex is not exact. About one in 1,500 to 2,000 babies are born with atypical genitalia. Then, doctors might designate a sex. Some intersex conditions remain undetected for years. These births illustrate the nonbinary nature of sex and gender.

15 What does "two-spirit" mean?

"Two-spirit" is used in some indigenous cultures to refer to someone who identifies with both masculine and feminine traits. This quality is revered in many tribes. Today, we might identify some two-spirit people as transgender, a much newer term.

Language

16 How does one respectfully refer to a transgender person?

The most respectful way to refer to a transgender person is by their name and pronouns. If you accidentally use the wrong pronoun, apologize and keep talking. "Transsexual" is considered to be dated and inaccurate. Use transgender as an adjective, but not as a noun, even if you hear some transgender people do that. Referring to someone as "a transgender" reduces a person's whole identity to one quality.

17 How does one ask a transgender or nonbinary person about their pronouns?

It is easy. Listen to see if people tell you their pronouns as they introduce themselves. By stating your own pronouns, you invite people to tell you theirs. "I'm Terry and my pronouns are she/her/hers." You can say "I want to make sure I use the right pronouns for you. What are your pronouns?" A sincere, respectful question is appreciated. If you are

Pronouns respondents ask people to use

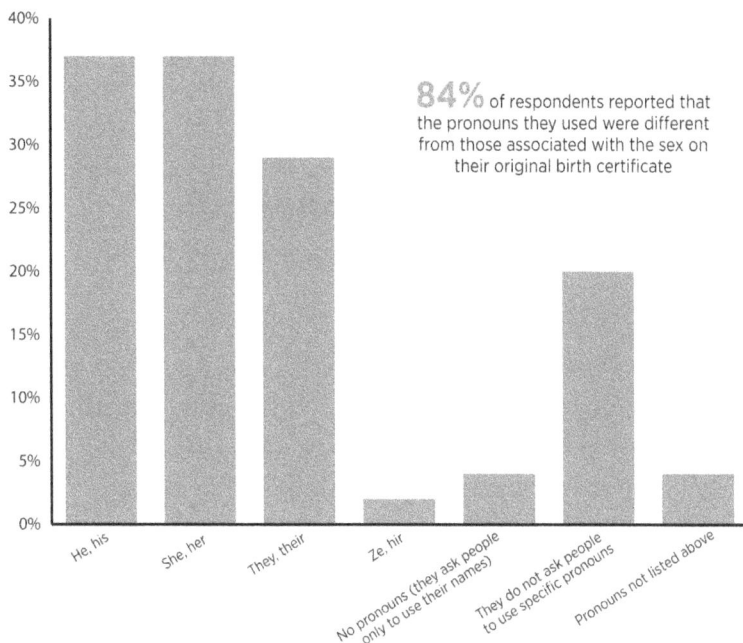

84% of respondents reported that the pronouns they used were different from those associated with the sex on their original birth certificate

Source: U.S. Transgender Survey

Graphic by Kacy Kobakof

introducing someone and know their pronouns, you can use one in your introduction: "This is my friend Kelly. They work in finance."

18 Why is there lack of agreement on terms such as LGBT?

Different groups use different letters in different arrangements. There is no consensus. The issue is that there are many identities and orientations under the umbrella and, historically, not all were recognized or included. There is not a wrong way to use the letters as long as it is with respectful knowledge that the group is very diverse. In this guide, for consistency, we will generally use LGBTQ+. The + signifies that there are more possibilities.

19 Why do many transgender people prefer not to be called "transgendered?"

Using -ed after the word transgender turns it into a passive verb. It implies that something occurred that caused the person's gender to change. More likely, it was miscategorized at birth. Individuals are in charge of their transitions. Being transgender is not something that happens to someone; it is who they are. It is better to say someone has transitioned.

20 Do some people prefer to be identified as men or women rather than with a trans- prefix?

It depends on context. Some people use the prefix to acknowledge their transition. Others prefer to simply be called a man or a woman because that is how they identify. In most work and social contexts, identity is either known or not relevant to the conversation. Then, the prefix is not needed.

21 Is it OK to ask a person if they have had surgery or hormone therapy?

No. It is an invasion of privacy to ask anyone medical questions. This is especially true with gender changes, which are varied and intimate. For transgender people, questions like this can be triggers to identity struggles and cause long periods of distress. Many transgender people, most of whom have never had surgery, feel that the question challenges their identity or authenticity.

History

22 Are transgender identities new?

No. There are centuries-old descriptions of transgender or nonbinary people and identities in Africa, Asia, Europe and North and South America. Some people were accorded sacred significance. Others were shunned or persecuted and their stories suppressed. Although the transgender identity is not new, visibility and acceptance in the United States are new.

23 When did the U.S. transgender rights movement begin?

In the 1940s, Louise Lawrence developed a network of transgender people centered in San Francisco. Part of that network founded the publication "Transvestia: The Journal of the American Society for Equality in Dress" in 1952. Around then, American-born Christine Jorgensen returned to the United States after gender-confirming surgery in Denmark. She spoke out for transgender rights. In 1969, transgender people including Sylvia Rivera, Marsha P. Johnson and Miss Major Griffin-Gracy played key roles in the Stonewall uprising in New York.

24 Why is Christine Jorgensen important to the transgender movement?

Jorgensen, an ex-soldier from New York City, brought the issue of gender identity to national attention. She overcame widespread and inaccurate press accounts to become a spokeswoman for transgender people. Jorgensen told her story through the press, on stage and on campuses. In many ways, she was the first person to publicly validate and describe gender transition.

25 What is the Stonewall uprising?

The Stonewall Inn was a LGBTQ+ nightclub in Greenwich Village raided by police on June 28, 1969. Raids at such clubs were not unusual in the 1960s. This raid escalated into rioting, and protests followed. The following June, pride parades were held in memory of Stonewall. In more recent years, some activists have said the role of transgender people at Stonewall has been minimized.

26 When were national organizations for transgender rights created?

The National Transgender Advocacy Coalition, a lobbying group, was founded in 1999. It was started because groups that supported similar interests did not always include transgender rights in their lobbying efforts. In 2002, the Transgender Law Center started in Oakland, California. In 2003, the National Center for Transgender Equality was founded in Washington, D.C.

27 Have transgender people been elected to political office?

There have been a few. Pioneers include:

- Joanne Conte, city councilwoman in Arvada, Colorado, elected in 1991
- Althea Gaines, Republican elected to the Massachusetts House in 1992
- Jessica Orsini, alderwoman, Centralia, Missouri, 2006
- Stu Rasmussen, mayor of Silverton, Oregon, elected in 2008
- Victoria Kolakowski, Alameda County Superior Court judge, elected in 2010
- Danica Roem, Democrat, Virginia House, elected in 2017

28 How is transgender history being made today?

The situation remains fluid in research, coalition building, legislation and the courts. In October 2016, the U.S. Supreme Court accepted the case of a transgender student who asked to use the boys' restroom in his Virginia high school. The case grew out of guidance from the Obama administration's Departments of Education and Justice. The letter said federal law required local schools to "treat transgender students consistent with their gender identity." However, in February 2017, the new Trump administration rescinded the letter and, in March, the Supreme Court said it would not hear the case and sent it back to the lower court.

Coming Out

29 How do people decide when they should come out?

It depends. This can be a long process of reflecting on one's experiences and feelings. According to the U.S. Transgender Survey, almost 60 percent of people who come out as transgender do so between the ages of 16 and 25. For many, coming out is gradual and does not happen all at once. Transgender people who do not come out are still transgender. Coming out does not make identity more valid.

30 What are key parts of the process?

Coming out begins by accepting oneself. That is usually followed by coming out to one group. That could mean friends, family or coworkers. The order depends on what is safest and most comfortable. Some come out only to certain people. Some people have come out and been pressured to detransition. They might later decide to try again.

Negative Experiences Among Transgender People

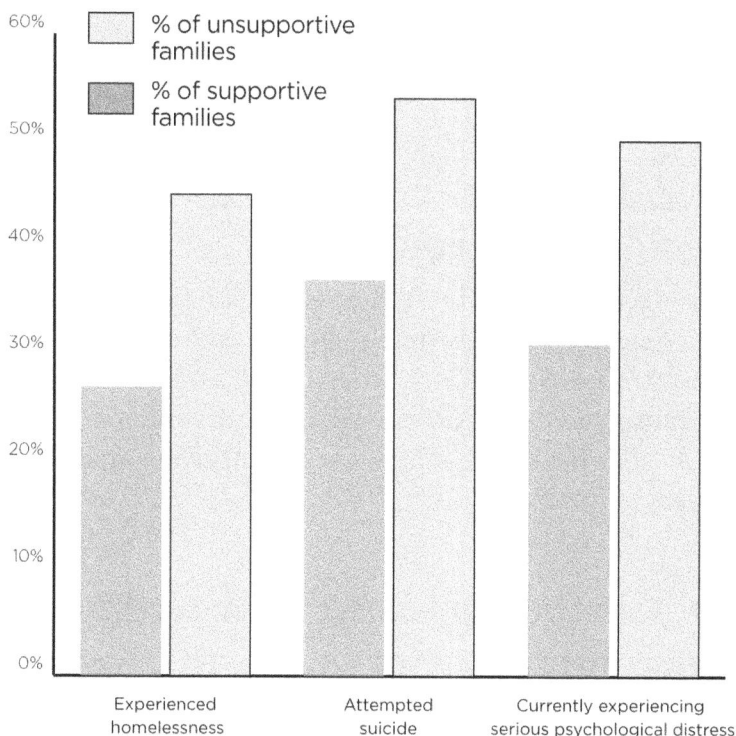

60%

☐ % of unsupportive families

■ % of supportive families

50%

40%

30%

20%

10%

0%

Experienced homelessness

Attempted suicide

Currently experiencing serious psychological distress

Source: U.S. Transgender Survey

Graphic by Terri Powys

31 How do transgender people know when others are receptive?

Transgender people don't always know if others will accept their identity. Signs from family and friends can help people decide to come out. Many people prepare by thinking about what to say, forming a support group and accepting the possibility of negative reactions. Carefully choosing the moment and way to tell can help. Coming out is ongoing, as people must decide whether to disclose when they meet new people or change jobs or schools. The Human Rights Campaign calls this ongoing process "living openly."

32 Do some transgender people decide not to come out?

Yes. According to GLAAD, it can sometimes feel disempowering for people to disclose they are transgender. Sometimes, when others learn someone is transgender, they do not accept their gender as real and valid. In some countries, it is dangerous or even illegal to be transgender.

33 Is there pressure from within the community for people to come out?

According to GLAAD, some transgender and nonbinary people publicly discuss their lives to raise awareness and encourage others to live openly. Some want others to come out, too. Those who do not disclose that they are transgender are said to be passing or living stealth transgender lives. This has led to situations in which people feel shamed into coming out.

Myths and Stereotypes

34 Children can't really understand gender, can they?

Yes, they can. Children under the age of 5 have shown signs that their sex assigned at birth does not match their identity. However, the signs are not always recognized or acknowledged by parents and doctors. Sometimes, the signs are ignored.

35 Are people really transgender if they do not get surgery or hormone treatments?

Yes, they really are. Being transgender has to do with gender identity, not with what genitalia a person has. Questioning this can challenge a person's identity and authenticity.

36 Are transgender people drag kings and queens or crossdressers?

Drag is performance art that is done for live shows. It is not necessarily the way one identifies in everyday life. Performing in drag does not mean a person is transgender, though some transgender people do drag. Crossdressing is when people wear clothing or accessories of another gender, often in private. This alone does not make them transgender. The terms transvestite and transvestism are outdated and may offend.

37 How many people who transition later want to reverse the change?

Eight percent of the people in the U.S. Transgender Survey said they detransitioned. Reasons they reported for the reversal included harassment, trouble finding work and pressure from a parent, spouse or family members. For about two-thirds of that 8 percent, the reversal was temporary.

38 What is "sex-change regret?"

This is the belief that many people who transition regret having the surgery and want to have it reversed or take their lives. There are stories about this on the Internet and some books about it. Some cite research. However, newer research debunks this. While transitioning is not without difficulties, recent research shows that few people detransition and that transitioning actually reduces suicides.

39 Are racial minority families less accepting of gender transition?

The 2011 Transgender Discrimination Survey results disputed that, despite evidence that minority trans people are generally subject to more discrimination. The survey showed that Black, Asian, Native American and Latino families had slightly higher rates than White families of accepting transgender members. The 2015 survey found that almost all racial groups had acceptance rates of about 50 percent.

Media

40 Do news media portray transgender people accurately?

According to GLAAD, founded by media professionals, coverage should be better. It issued a report in 2013 after the transition of soldier Chelsea Manning, who had been convicted of violating the Espionage Act. She received clemency in 2017. GLAAD reported, "The media has a long and poor track record of reporting on transgender people … The coverage that we have seen thus far has relied on stereotypical images, contrived confusion over names and pronouns, and an obsession with surgery." Other critics have called for more coverage of violence against transgender people, and some want to see more positive stories. They wanted less of a focus on physical changes.

41 What would make news coverage more accurate?

GLAAD's media reference guide has several suggestions for covering the transgender community. They include:

- Learn and use basic terms, respect name and pronoun wishes and avoid offensive terms.
- Move beyond coming-out stories to leadership issues.
- Focus on more than medical issues and don't refer to being transgender as a mental disorder.
- Cover hate violence, discrimination and poverty but also include mainstream transgender people in general stories.

42 How are transgender people portrayed on television?

GLAAD examined primetime broadcast network series, cable networks and streaming services for the 2016-2017 TV season. In many cases, it considered all LGBTQ+ coverage together. It found:

- On scripted primetime broadcast programming, 4.8 percent of characters were identified as gay, lesbian, bisexual, transgender or queer. This was the highest percentage of LGBTQ+ series regulars GLAAD had ever reported. Twenty-eight characters were recurring.
- Three transgender characters were counted on broadcast, six on cable and seven on streaming original series. This was up from seven the year before. Four were identified as men.

43 Do transgender roles typically go to cisgender actors?

Historically, transgender characters were played solely by cisgender actors. This is changing. Transgender actress Jen Richards said hiring cisgender people to play transgender roles denies transgender people opportunities and does not allow for fully authentic performances. She has said that audiences reward cisgender actors for playing transgender roles, while transgender people get punished for living their real truth.

44 How do social media platforms allow users to declare their gender identity?

Social media have been adding options beyond male and female. In 2014, Facebook added 50 options for gender identity. They included transgender, bigender, gender fluid, gender-nonconforming and two-spirit. Dating sites such as Tinder and OkCupid also have added options for gender identity.

Families

45 How do families react when a member transitions?

This varies, even within families. According to the U.S. Transgender Survey, 60 percent of respondents said they found support in their immediate families. However, 10 percent said that a family member had become violent in response to their transition. Eight percent said they had been kicked out of their homes, and 10 percent said they ran away. Generally, people who transitioned at older ages reported more rejection. Twenty-one percent of parents who came out to their families as transgender said at least one of their children stopped talking to them.

46 Do family relationships later improve?

In the 2011 National Transgender Discrimination Survey, 61 percent said relationships improved after they came out. Furthermore, 45 percent said their family was as strong as it had been before they came out. The greatest improvement was for Black and Asian respondents and people without high school diplomas.

47 How do spouses and partners react?

In the U.S. Transgender Survey, more than one fourth of respondents said they had lost a relationship with their partner after coming out. Breakups were more likely for people who transitioned or who came out at older ages. Furthermore, this happened twice more frequently with transgender women than with transgender men.

48 Do transgender people have children of their own?

Certainly, though it is related to age. Fourteen percent of the people in the U.S. Transgender Survey said they had a related child under age 18 living in their households. Nationally, about 34 percent of all U.S. adults said so, according to the Current Population Survey.

49 How important is family support to transgender people?

According to PFLAG's "Our Trans Loved Ones," research shows family support is vital to mental and physical wellbeing for transgender and gender-expansive young people. The organization's site offers family support, resources and an online academy. It has chapters in almost every state for families and friends who want to learn more and be supportive.

50 How can parents support children who transition?

There is no short answer for this and every family is different. PFLAG and the Family Acceptance Project at San Francisco State University are starting points. The resource section in the back of this guide has more. It points to material for people of different ages, races, languages and religions.

When a Spouse/Partner is Most Likely to End a Relationship

The age at which a respondent transitioned also affected the likelihood of a relationship ending. Respondents who transitioned at age 35 or older were more than twice as likely to experience the end of a relationship solely due to being transgender (24%).

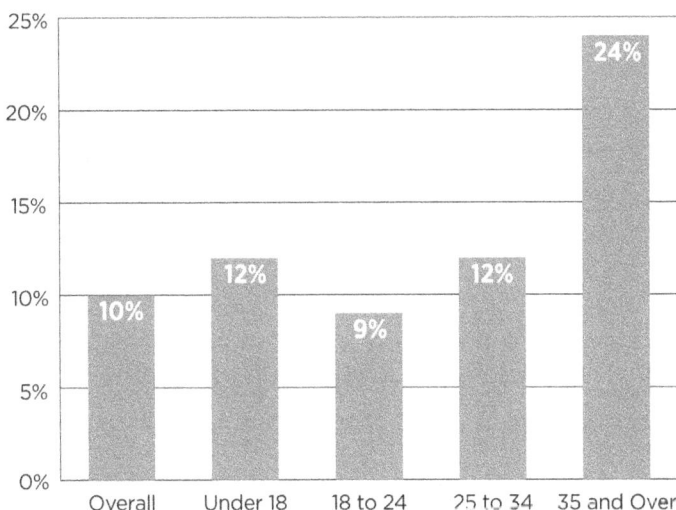

	Overall	Under 18	18 to 24	25 to 34	35 and Over
	10%	12%	9%	12%	24%

Source: US Transgender Survey   Graphic by Kathleen Kennedy

Acceptance

51 How accepting is U.S. society overall of transgender rights?

This varies by issue and age, among other things. Major issues include employment and health care. The 2015 U.S. Transgender Survey found that 68 percent of respondents said co-workers accepted them. That was greater acceptance than they reported among family members or at school. A 2016 Reuters/Ipsos opinion poll on public restrooms found greater acceptance among younger people. The poll found that Americans aged 18-29 were twice as likely to support letting people use restrooms that corresponded with their identity. People 60 and older were twice as likely to want people to follow the sex on their birth certificate.

52 Are transgender people accepted more or less than gay people?

Gay people are more accepted, according to surveys, but transgender acceptance is catching up. After the Reuters/Ipsos results were released, the Christian

Science Monitor reported that acceptance was growing faster for transgender people than it had for gays and lesbians. Knowing an individual can be key. A Pew study in August and September of 2016 found that 87 percent of people knew someone who is gay or lesbian. Just three in 10 said they knew someone who is transgender.

53 Are transgender people supported within the larger LGBTQ+ community?

Transgender author and activist Janet Mock said "The T is no longer going to be silent." Others have picked up that statement to illustrate that the LGBTQ+ movement has not always supported transgender people in legislation and legal actions. On some issues, transgender advocacy was seen as a barrier to getting new laws passed. Several national organizations have broadened their positions. Some have changed their names to include transgender people. But representation is still an issue.

54 Who are some influential openly transgender or binary people?

Kye Allums became the first openly transgender athlete in NCAA Division 1 when he played on the women's basketball team at George Washington University in 2010. He was designated female at birth but identifies as male.

Alexis Arquette appeared in dozens of movies, her most popular being "The Wedding Singer" in 1998.

Chaz Bono, son of Sonny and Cher, documented his transition in the 2012 film "Becoming Chaz."

Wendy Carlos scored music for films including "The Shining" and "A Clockwork Orange." Her "Switched-On Bach," became one of the first classical music albums to sell 500,000 copies.

Carmen Carreras is a model, reality TV actress and burlesque performer.

Laverne Cox stars on the web TV series "Orange is the New Black." She was the first transgender person to be nominated for a Primetime Emmy. Cox appeared on the cover of the May 2014 TIME magazine issue that declared a "transgender tipping point."

Laura Jane Grace, whose band, Against Me! released the album "Transgender Dysphoria Blues."

Harisu, a K-pop star and actress in South Korea, changed her gender in the 1990s.

Caitlyn Jenner, who won an Olympic gold medal as a man, received heavy media attention when she came out as transgender in 2015. While this raised visibility, some argue her story was sensationalized and did not represent the community well.

Jazz Jennings stars in her own TLC show "I am Jazz." The show follows the life of Jazz and her family as she transitions. She also wrote "Being Jazz: My Life as a (Transgender) Teen."

Lana Lawless went to court to win removal of the

requirement that golfers in the Ladies Professional Golf Association be designated female at birth.

Janet Mock published a best-selling memoir about her transition, "Redefining Realness," and hosted an MSNBC web talk show about pop culture.

Chris Mosier became the first openly transgender member of Team USA and competed at the Duathlon World Championships in Spain. He then became the first transgender athlete in a Nike ad.

Ataru Nakamura, a Japanese pop music idol, has been writing, recording and performing since she was 14.

Renee Richards won a 1977 ruling by the New York Supreme Court to compete in tennis tournaments as a transgender woman.

Jacob Tobia is a performer, Internet personality, writer, producer and advocate for nonbinary, genderqueer, and gender nonconforming people.

Alok Vaid-Menon is a gender non-conforming writer, poet, entertainer and performance artist.

Lilly and **Lana Wachowski**, who produced the Matrix trilogy as the Wachowski brothers, both transitioned.

Jin Xing, once a male colonel in the Chinese army, now attracts 100 million viewers a week to her TV talk show.

55 What can institutions do to support transgender people?

It depends on the institution, of course. Initiatives can include gender-inclusive or nondiscriminatory policies and benefits. These will vary among companies, nonprofits, government agencies and schools. It helps to involve transgender members of the organization and transgender advocacy groups in assessing needs and creating policy.

56 How can people show acceptance?

Transgender people face a lack of understanding. Allies can narrow this gap by learning more and asking others to be more accepting as well. Asking transgender people to describe the issues they deal with helps. Some allies become advocates, supporting transgender people in their quest for acceptance and civil rights.

Religion

57 Are transgender people religious?

In the U.S. Transgender Survey, 19 percent of respondents who said they had been part of a spiritual or religious community also said they left because they were rejected. Forty-two percent of the people who left said they were welcomed into other spiritual or religious communities. Sixty-three percent said they were spiritual or religious. The remaining 37 percent said they were not. A 2014 Pew Research survey indicated that 23 percent of all Americans were religiously unaffiliated.

58 Which religious groups accept transgender people?

In 2015, the Pew Research Center offered a four-part breakdown:

Official statement of inclusion

- Episcopal Church
- Reform Judaism
- Unitarian Universalist Association
- United Church of Christ

Inclusion, no official statement

- Evangelical Lutheran Church in America
- Presbyterian Church (U.S.A.)
- United Methodist Church

Mixed or no official position

- African Methodist Episcopal Church
- Church of God (Cleveland, Tennessee)
- Presbyterian Church in America
- Roman Catholic Church

Stated barriers to inclusion

- Assemblies of God
- Church of Jesus Christ of Latter-Day Saints (Mormon)
- Lutheran Church-Missouri Synod
- Southern Baptist Convention

Religious or Spiritual Identities of Transgender Community

Current religious or spiritual identity	% of respondents
Spiritual, but no religious affiliation	25%
Agnostic	23%
Atheist	22%
Christian	21%
Pagan	9%
Buddhist	6%
Jewish	4%
Secular Humanist	4%
Wiccan	4%
Druid	1%
Hindu	1%
Muslim	1%
Native American Traditional Practitioner or Ceremonial	1%
Polytheist (write-in response)	1%
Taoist	1%
Baha'i	<1%
Confucian	<1%
Jain	<1%
Jehovah's Witness	<1%
Rastafarian	<1%
Scientologist	<1%
Shinto	<1%
Sikh	<1%
Tenrikyo	<1%
A religious affiliation or spiritual identity not listed above	7%
No affiliation	13%

Source: U.S. Transgender Survey
Graphic by Tori Zackery

59 What are churches' main issues with transgender people?

Some are reflected in church policies. The Methodist Church, facing a schism over whether LGBTQ+ people could be clergy, saw more than 100 clergy members come out. The Presbyterian Church (U.S.A.) and the Evangelical Lutheran Church in America have allowed ordinations of transgender people. Some evangelical churches advise clergy to counsel people to seek treatment. The Pentecostal denomination Assemblies of God discourages "any and all attempts to physically change, alter, or disagree with their predominant biological sex." The Southern Baptist Convention has said that transgender people must repent before they can join. The Mormon Church says people considering "elective transsexual operations" may not be baptized or confirmed. Those who have transitioned must seek approval. The Roman Catholic Church says the gender determined at birth is permanent. It says that people who have had procedures to change their gender are not allowed to marry in the church.

60 How is religion used to deny services and jobs to transgender people?

This is allowed under religious exemptions in state "religious freedom" or "employment nondiscrimination" acts. These cite First Amendment protections of religious organizations and businesses. Exemptions hold that employers cannot be forced to employ gay, lesbian, bisexual and transgender people. The exemption can apply even for jobs that do not serve a religious function.

Leaving a Faith Community Due to Rejection

YEARS SINCE TRANSITIONING (%)

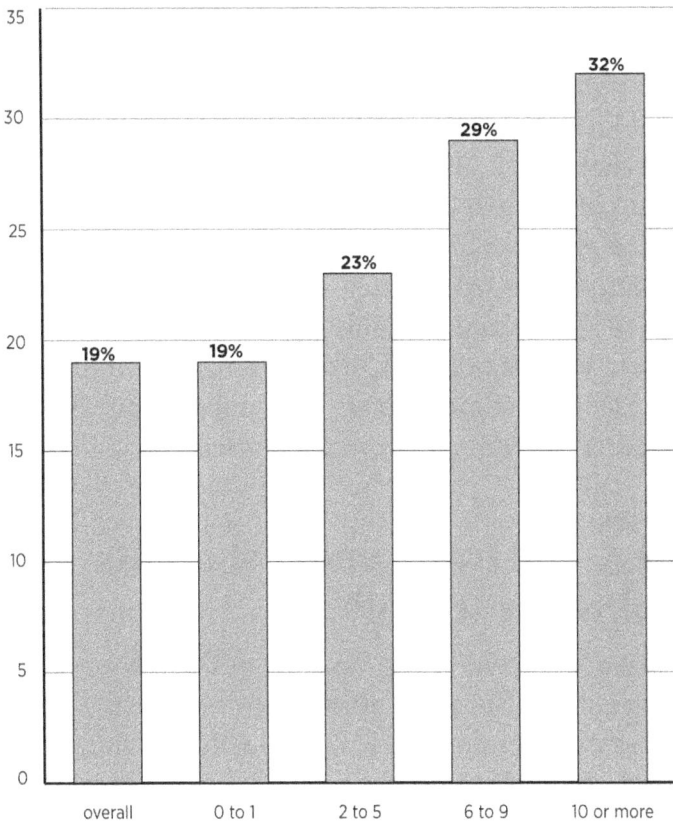

Source: U.S. Transgender Survey   Graphic by Emily Elconin

School

61 Does the federal Title IX cover the civil rights of transgender students?

This has changed 180 degrees. In March 2016, the Obama administration said the 1972 law protects the rights of transgender students to use restrooms and locker rooms that align with their gender. In February 2017, the Trump administration rescinded that guidance. It cited insufficient legal analysis and significant litigation. Trump had said the issue should be left up to states. Education Secretary Betsy DeVos said that although the guidance was rescinded, schools still have an obligation to protect transgender students from bullying and harassment. Further developments were expected.

62 Are transgender students bullied at school?

Fifty-six percent of respondents in the U.S. Transgender Survey reported they had been verbally harassed in grades K-12. One fourth said they had been physically attacked and 13 percent reported sexual assault. Twenty-four percent said they were targeted for aggression in post-secondary education.

Harassment in Schools

Percent of students that left K-12 school due to mistreatment

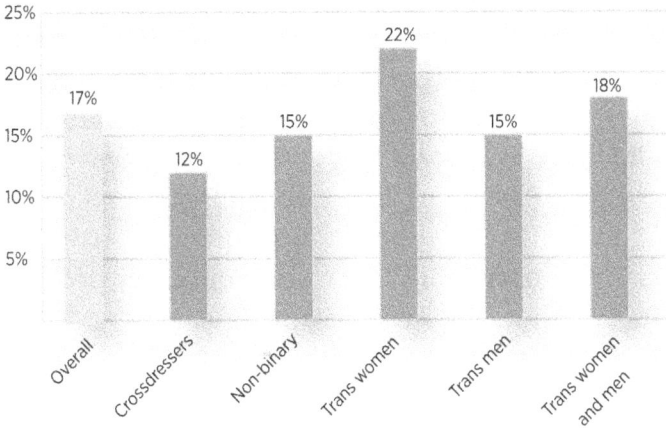

Source: US Transgender Survey　　　　　Graphic by: Eli Pales

Harassment in Higher Education

Percent of students that left college or vocational school
due to mistreatment

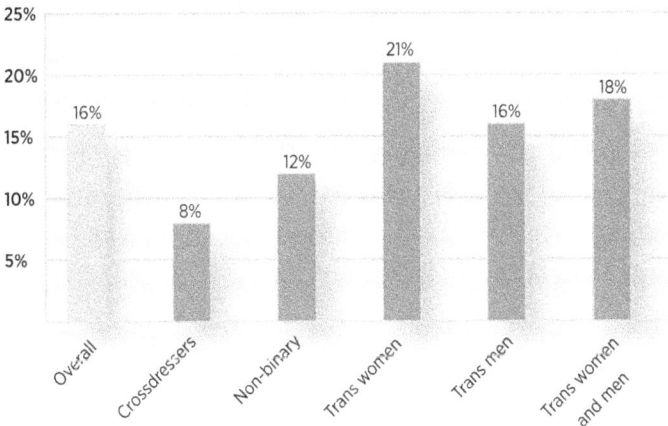

Source: US Transgender Survey　　　　　Graphic by: Eli Pales

63 How does bullying affect schoolchildren?

Bullying can lead to school absences and sickness. According to a National Education Association report, bullying makes transgender schoolchildren feel anxious, depressed and even suicidal. All children targeted for bullying and rejection are more likely to abuse illegal drugs and engage in risky sexual behavior. The U.S. Transgender Survey found that 22 percent of transgender women and 15 percent of transgender men and nonbinary people had left school because of aggression.

64 What services do colleges provide for transgender students?

Some colleges have created gender-inclusive housing options and appropriate restrooms. Transgender students have asked schools to make it easier for them to change their names and gender markers across academic records. They have asked for gender identity training for faculty, counselors and health providers. More inclusive insurance has also been suggested. Some have asked for help getting into and succeeding in college to overcome obstacles experienced in K-12 schools.

65 What are gender-inclusive housing options?

This can mean on-campus or community living according to or regardless of gender identity. It can mean having roommates who respect and accept their identities. More than 200 colleges and universities have such options to varying degrees.

Work

66 Is it more difficult for transgender people to get jobs?

Transgender and nonbinary people responding to the U.S. Transgender Survey reported an unemployment level of 15 percent. That was triple the level in the overall adult population. Joblessness is higher still for people who are both transgender and members of demographic groups with high unemployment. More than 26 percent of transgender people reported losing a job because of their identity.

67 What are income levels like for transgender people?

More than twice as many transgender people live in poverty compared to the general population, 29 percent vs. 14 percent, according to the 2015 survey. Twelve percent of transgender people said they had been homeless in the prior year. Thirty percent said they had been homeless at some point in their lives.

Individual and Household Income

Individual and household incomes for USTS sample and
U.S. population (Current Population Survey)

Individual Income in 2014

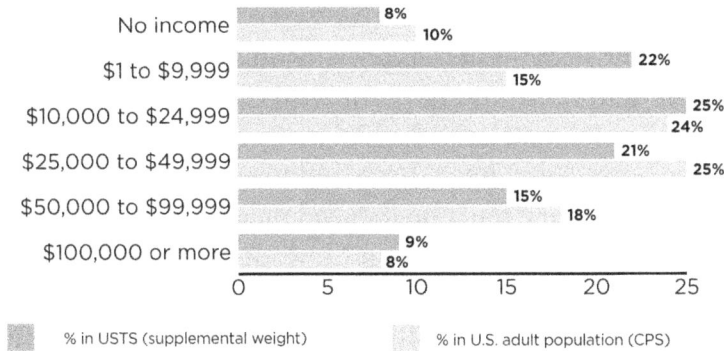

Income	% in USTS	% in U.S.
No income	8%	10%
$1 to $9,999	22%	15%
$10,000 to $24,999	25%	24%
$25,000 to $49,999	21%	25%
$50,000 to $99,999	15%	18%
$100,000 or more	9%	8%

■ % in USTS (supplemental weight)   ■ % in U.S. adult population (CPS)

Household Income in 2014

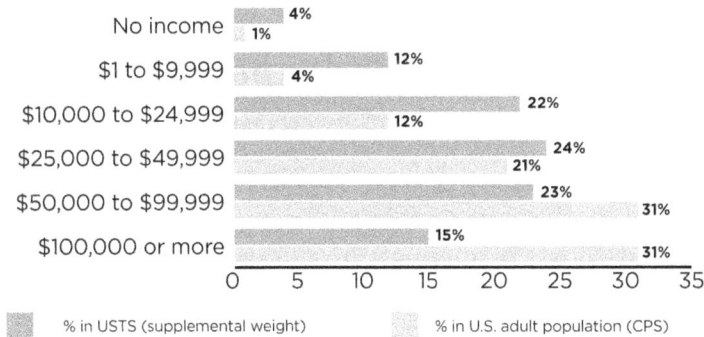

Income	% in USTS	% in U.S.
No income	4%	1%
$1 to $9,999	12%	4%
$10,000 to $24,999	22%	12%
$25,000 to $49,999	24%	21%
$50,000 to $99,999	23%	31%
$100,000 or more	15%	31%

■ % in USTS (supplemental weight)   ■ % in U.S. adult population (CPS)

Source: 2015 U.S. Transgender Survey   Graphic by Laura Bohannon

68 What is U.S. military policy about transgender people?

On Aug. 25, 2017, President Donald Trump directed the Pentagon to ban transgender individuals from openly serving in the U.S. armed forces. The order stopped the hiring of transgender military personnel. It also gave the Department of Defense latitude in deciding whether those already in the military could continue to serve. This reversed a 2016 Obama administration decision that would have allowed them to serve and have medical care, surgery and name and gender changes in the Pentagon's personnel system. Trump had tweeted in July 2017, "Our military must be focused on decisive and overwhelming victory and cannot be burdened with the tremendous medical costs and disruption that transgender in the military would entail." At the time, an estimated 6,000 transgender people were already in the military.

69 Do transgender people work in the underground economy?

Some do. Twenty percent said in the U.S. Transgender Survey that at some point in their lives they had made income with illegal activities. These included selling drugs and other criminal acts. Nineteen percent said they had done sex work for money, food or a place to sleep.

Current and Past Military Service

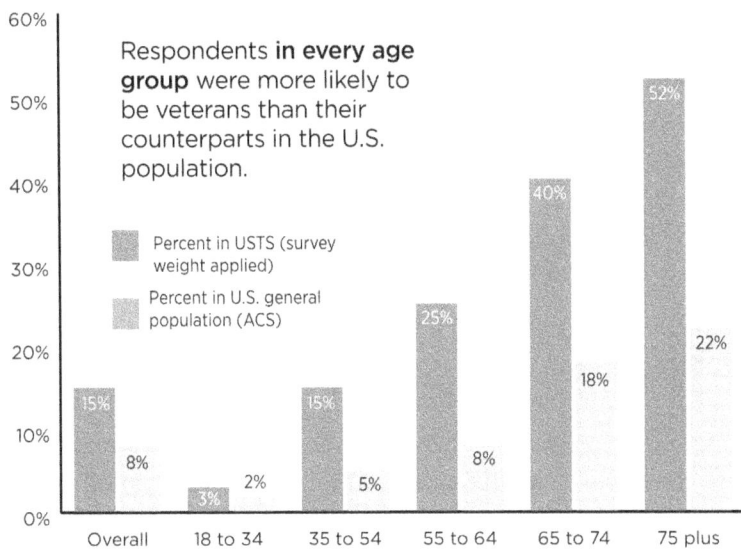

Respondents **in every age group** were more likely to be veterans than their counterparts in the U.S. population.

Percent in USTS (survey weight applied)

Percent in U.S. general population (ACS)

	Overall	18 to 34	35 to 54	55 to 64	65 to 74	75 plus
USTS	15%	3%	15%	25%	40%	52%
ACS	8%	2%	5%	8%	18%	22%

Source: U.S. Transgender Survey   Graphic by McKenna Ross

Health

70 Does being transgender constitute having a mental illness?

In 2012, the Diagnostic and Statistical Manual of Mental Disorders that is widely used in the United State changed this. Having a transgender identity went from being diagnosed with "Gender identity disorder" to "Gender dysphoria." This allowed people to get a diagnosis, treatment and care without the stigma of having a disorder.

71 What is gender dysphoria?

According to the American Psychiatric Association, this "involves a conflict between a person's physical gender and the gender with which he or she identifies." A similar diagnostic change was made for sexual orientation in 1973. Gender dysphoria can mean stress, anxiety and depression related to gender identity. Dysphoria does not mean gender nonconformity. It is anxiety about thoughts, feelings and behaviors that do not match stereotypes of the sex assigned at birth. Not all transgender people have gender dysphoria.

72 Does transitioning affect mental health?

Social and medical transitioning can decrease the disconnect between sex and gender and greatly improve mental health. Transitioning can also mean changes in relationships with family, friends and significant others. Most people report improvements. Transition can also bring new challenges in stigma, discrimination and assault. There can be disappointment that transitioning does not bring as much improvement as was anticipated. For all, mental health is an ongoing process that takes work and help.

73 What is hormone therapy?

This is adding or inhibiting hormones. The most common are testosterone for transmasculine people and estrogen for transfeminine people. These can help achieve desired physical characteristics and a psychological state that matches gender identity. Although 78 percent of respondents in the U.S. Transgender Survey wanted hormone treatment, only 49 percent ever received it. Finances and insurance can be barriers. About 10 percent of people who use hormones get them from unlicensed sources such as friends and the Internet.

74 What is gender-confirming surgery?

There are many surgeries that transgender people can undergo as part of their transition. A transgender person can have none, some, or several of them. For transgender women, gender-confirming surgery can include breast augmentation and vaginoplasty. For transgender men, the most common are chest reconstruction and hysterectomies.

75 What is the medical cost of transitioning?

In 2015, CNN cited the Philadelphia Center for Transgender Surgery as saying it can cost as much as $140,450 to transition from male to female. Transition from female to male was $124,400. Remember that most transgender people do not get surgery and that there are different degrees to which someone can go.

76 Does health insurance cover gender transition?

Not always. Some health-care providers still categorize some procedures as cosmetic and will not cover them. There are three ways that people commonly receive health insurance: employer-provided plans, government-subsidized plans and state health plans. Complete coverage of transgender-related care varies from state to state and plan to plan.

Trouble with Insurance

Transgender patients have trouble getting care covered

Negative insurance action	% of respondents who reported insurance action
Denied coverage for transition-related surgery	55%
Covered only some of the surgical care needed for transition	42%
Denied coverage for transition-related hormone therapy	25%
Covered surgery for transition, but had no surgery providers in their network	21%
Refused to change records to list current name or gender	17%
Denied coverage for care often considered gender-specific due to transgender status	13%
Denied other routine health care because of transgender status	7%

Source: U.S. Transgender Survey   Graphic by Eli Pales

77 What is the suicide rate for transgender people?

Suicidal thoughts and behaviors are much higher among transgender people than for the U.S. population overall. The suicide attempt rate for the total population is 4.6 percent, according to the 2015 National Survey on Drug Use and Health. The U.S. Transgender Survey uncovered a suicide attempt rate of 40 percent. When asked about suicidal ideation in the past year, the overall population had a 4 percent rate. This is in contrast to 48 percent among transgender people. Some factors led to even higher rates. Those included losing a job because of bias, school bullying, low income and physical or sexual assault. Suicide attempts are lower for people with steady work, higher income, stable housing and accepting families. However, even then rates are still much higher than for the general population.

78 What is conversion therapy?

Conversion therapy is a discredited and unethical treatment purported to change a person's sexual orientation or gender identity. It has been scientifically disproven. It can cause psychological distress and increase suicide attempts, running away and homelessness. According to the Movement Advancement Project, 45 states allow conversion therapy for minors. In the U.S. Transgender Survey, 14 percent said their immediate family had sent them to a therapist, counselor, or religious/spiritual adviser to try to prevent them from transitioning.

Attempted suicide in the past year

Current Age (%)

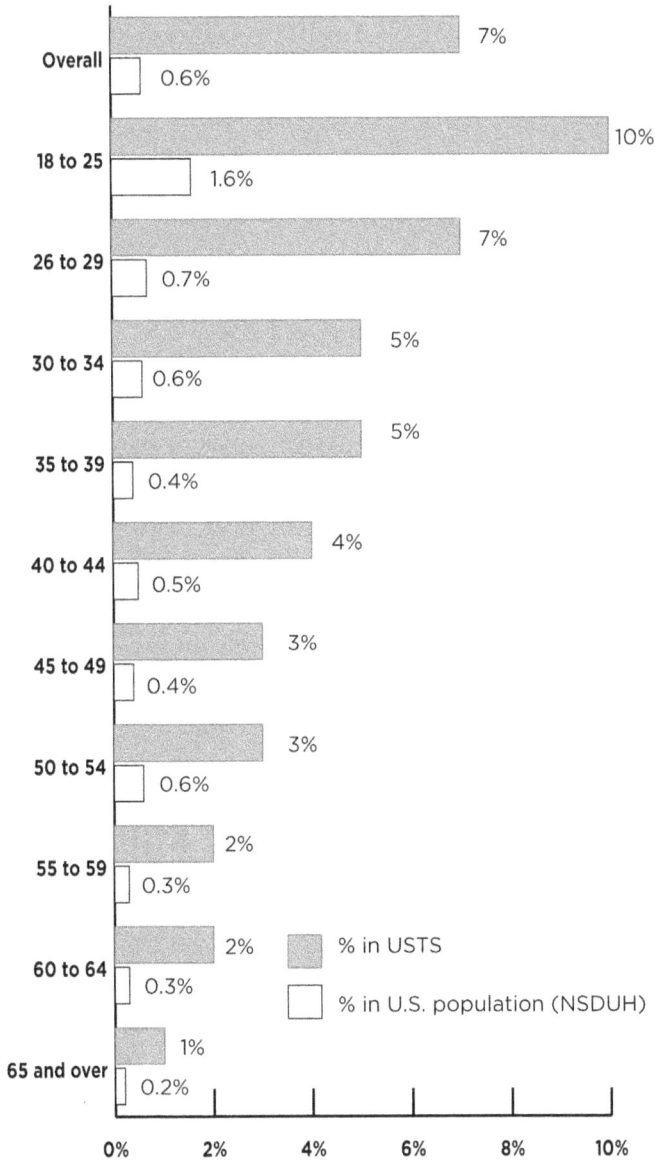

Age	% in USTS	% in U.S. population (NSDUH)
Overall	7%	0.6%
18 to 25	10%	1.6%
26 to 29	7%	0.7%
30 to 34	5%	0.6%
35 to 39	5%	0.4%
40 to 44	4%	0.5%
45 to 49	3%	0.4%
50 to 54	3%	0.6%
55 to 59	2%	0.3%
60 to 64	2%	0.3%
65 and over	1%	0.2%

Safety

79 Are transgender people targets of hate crimes?

Yes. The FBI reported 114 hate crimes over gender identity in 2015. This was almost four times the number from 2013, when such statistics were first tracked. Advocates say many crimes go unrecognized or unreported. Beyond hate crimes, the U.S. Transgender Survey revealed pervasive mistreatment. Forty-six percent of respondents said they have been verbally harassed and 9 percent reported being physically attacked. One in 10 reported having been sexually assaulted in the previous year. Nearly half said they had been sexually assaulted at some time in their lives.

80 Are people getting killed over their gender identity?

The number of documented transgender killings are at a record high in the United States. The Human Rights Campaign said advocates documented 21 homicides of transgender people in 2015. The Advocate publication reported 27 homicides in 2016. Homicides in 2017 were on pace to exceed those numbers. Nearly all the victims were Black or Hispanic women. Several studies have shown that hate crimes are higher for transgender women of color than for any other group.

81 Why is the risk greatest for transgender women of color?

Risks and disadvantages are compounded for people who belong to two or more marginalized groups. Non-White transgender women face greater challenges in safety, employment and other areas.

82 Is gender-identity violence an issue in other countries?

Transgender Europe has reported 2,016 killings of transgender and gender-diverse people worldwide in 2008-2015. Three-fourths were in Central and South America.

83 Have police been able to help?

Most respondents in the U.S. Transgender Survey, 57 percent, said they are uncomfortable asking police for help. Fifty-eight percent said police who suspected they were transgender had mistreated them.

84 Are transgender people stigmatized as victims?

Assaults and suicide have led to stigma, yes. While group statistics are real, projecting those numbers onto individuals is stereotyping. So is ignoring other aspects of transgender lives and focusing on just one or two dimensions. Learning about transgender people living happy, fulfilling lives completes the picture.

Civil Rights

85 Do transgender people have the same protections as gay people?

No. Rights vary based on state laws and local ordinances. In some cases, transgender people were not included in laws covering gay, lesbian and bisexual people. In other cases, transgender people were excluded specifically to help get legislation passed.

86 Are laws written to curtail transgender people's rights?

The Human Rights Coalition called 2016 a peak year for anti-transgender legislation. It reported that about 175 anti-transgender bills were filed. Most were about restrooms and public spaces. Two bills revolved around transgender marriage. The first required disclosure of previous "sex reassignment surgeries," and the second required that husbands and wives be natural-born men and women.

87 Do transgender people have marriage rights?

So far, yes. Some United States courts previously used the ban on gay marriage to ban transgender people from getting married. This included those who were straight but who had not or could not change their gender marker. The U.S. Supreme Court legalized same-sex marriage on June 26, 2015. This spurred efforts to outlaw marriage on the basis of gender transitions.

88 Are transgender people protected from workplace discrimination?

There is no national law protecting transgender people from workplace discrimination. However, 19 states have varying degrees of protection. More than 200 cities and counties have laws banning gender-identity discrimination. Local ordinances, charter provisions and executive orders from some governors also protect transgender rights.

Avoiding Anti-Transgender Discrimination

Respondents who held a job in the past year were asked a series of questions about actions they took in order to avoid discrimination at work in the past year, including hiding their gender identity, delaying their transition, and quitting their job. More than three-quarters (77%) took one or more actions to avoid discrimination. Respondents who were living in poverty (82%), non-binary respondents (81%), and people with disabilities (81%) were more likely to take one or more of these steps to avoid discrimination.

Actions taken to avoid anti-transgender discrimination at work in the past year	% of those who had a job
They had to hide their gender identity	53%
They did not ask employer to use pronouns they prefer (such as he, she or they)	47%
They delayed their gender transition	26%
They stayed in a job they would have preferred to leave	26%
They hid the fact that they had already transitioned gender	25%
They kept a job for which they were overqualified	24%
They quit their job	15%
They did not seek promotion or raise	13%
They requested transfer to a different position or department	6%
One or more experiences listed	**77%**

Source: US Transgender Survey   Graphic by Rachel Beard

Restrooms

89 Why has the restroom debate become so big?

At its root, this is not about restrooms, but civil rights and safety. The major argument against transgender people using public restrooms has been the myth that men dressing as women are a threat to women and children. There is no evidence that transgender people harass others in restrooms. In fact, public restrooms are where most sexual assaults against transgender people take place, according to the U.S. Transgender Survey. Early in 2017, eight states were considering restricted access to restrooms, locker rooms, and other sex-segregated facilities, according to the National Conference of State Legislatures. In July 2017, New Jersey adopted laws protecting people's right to choose restrooms or locker rooms that match their gender identity.

90 What was the significance of the 2016 North Carolina restroom bill?

On March 23, 2016, North Carolina became the first state to ban people from public restrooms and locker rooms that do not match the sex on their birth certificates. The law overturned local ordinances protecting LGBTQ+ people. Backlash and boycotts ensued. Forbes estimated that these cost North Carolina more than $600 million. Under this pressure, the state repealed the law on March 30, 2017. However, the state still prevented changes in local ordinances relating to private employment and public accommodation until 2020.

91 Which restroom do transgender people use?

Transgender people would like to use the restroom that best fits their gender identity. Outward appearance and surgical status have no bearing on a person's identity. Gender-inclusive or gender-free restrooms may be used by anyone.

92 Why do people need to use the restroom that aligns with their gender identity?

This is important for the mental health of transgender people, studies show. Being required to use a restroom that does not align with one's identity can be inappropriate and uncomfortable. It can raise self-doubts and it can be unsafe. Using a restroom that does not match expression has exposed people to violence. Twenty-six percent of transgender people reported being denied access or other problems in using the restrooms they want.

93 Do transgender people avoid using public restrooms?

The U.S. Transgender Survey found that 59 percent of respondents had avoided public restrooms in the previous year because they feared confrontation. Additionally, 31 percent limited drinking or meals to avoid needing to use public restrooms.

94 Would transgender restrooms help?

Gender-inclusive restrooms are for anyone. The designation of transgender restrooms is a problem. A transgender designation would out people who use it, putting them at risk. Another problem is that trans-exclusive restrooms might become the only option. Many transgender people just want to use a men's or women's room or one that is nonspecific.

Identity
Documents

95 What documents need to be changed when a person transitions?

Many documents include gender or sex. First, transgender people have to change the name and sex on their birth certificate. After this, it's common to change driver's licenses and Social Security cards. Gender or sex is noted on records for work, school, banks, credit applications, insurance, property deeds, immigration papers, passports, airline tickets and more.

96 Have most transgender people updated their IDs?

According to the U.S. Transgender Survey, 11 percent of respondents said all their documents had their new gender identity and name. Sixty-eight percent said none of their documents did.

97 How much does it cost to update IDs?

In the U.S. Transgender Survey, 35 percent said cost had been a barrier. Thirty-four percent reported spending more than $250 for a name change, and 11 percent spent more than $500. That does not include other documents.

98 Must transgender people provide proof of surgery to get new documents?

State laws and company policies vary. Some make it easy. The most burdensome rules require a court order or proof of surgery. The National Center for Transgender Equality has a state-by-state guide to requirements.

99 Can outdated IDs be a problem?

An ID that does not match gender presentation can reveal someone is transgender. This can happen when cashing a check, at a bar or in a traffic stop. The U.S. Transgender Survey found that 32 percent of respondents were harassed or denied benefits or service when caught in this situation. Nine percent were asked to leave establishments. Two percent said they were assaulted or attacked. These incidents were down about a third from results in the 2011 National Transgender Survey.

Experiences Updating Name on Specific IDs

The chart reflects respondents who have been able to update some or all of their IDs only omitting those who have not been able to update any IDs. It also does not include those who do not have the ID/record or do not want to update it. These numbers should not be reported without clearly stating that they represent only a subset of the respondents.

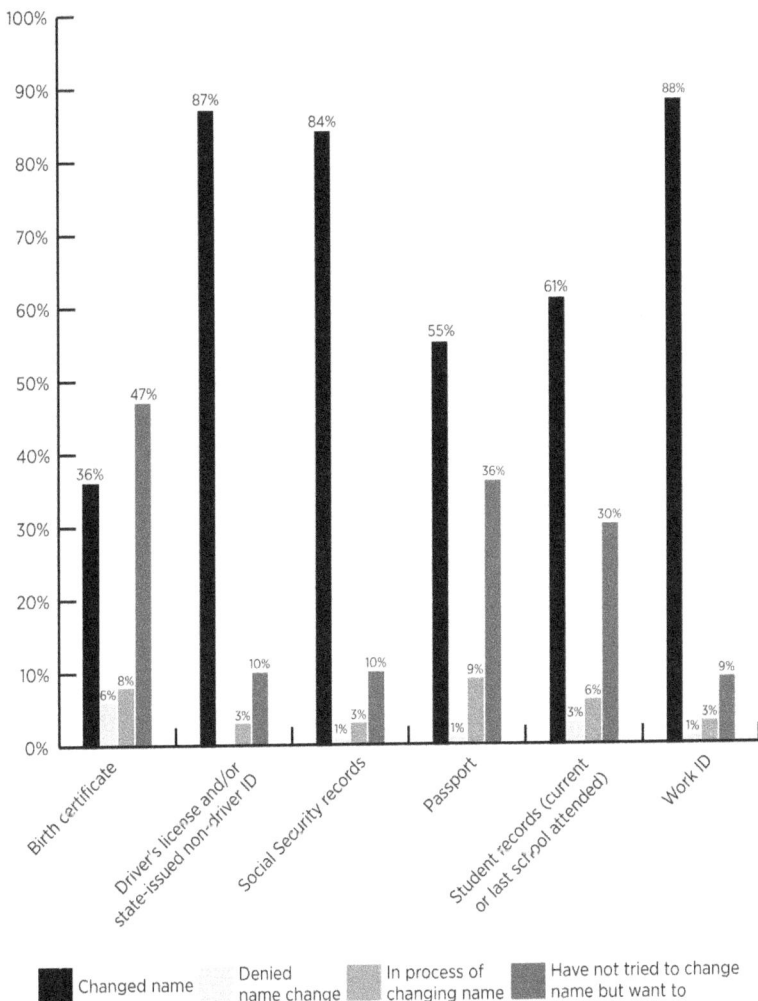

Changed name
Denied name change
In process of changing name
Have not tried to change name but want to

100 What is wrong with forms that ask "male" or "female"?

Checking "male" or "female" is fine if you identify as one or the other and never transition. However, it is a problem for people who are nonbinary or who transition. Nonbinary and genderqueer people call the two-box system "erasure" that implies their identity does not exist.

Epilogue

Hours before the last meeting of the journalism class that wrote this guide, the National Center for Transgender Equality released the largest ever study of transgender and nonbinary people. We had been advised by the center to wait for that survey, and its release sharpened our guide. The key question after reading a large study like the U.S. Transgender Survey or a small guide like this one is what to do with the information. Two answers came at the press conference when the report was released.

Survey Project Manager Sandy E. James said, "It's very important for people to stop making it seem like trans people are various people over there ... Trans people are your neighbors. They're in school with you. They're not some phenomenon that people read about in books." This report "should be an educational piece for everyone. It's not just for policy makers. It's for your parents. It's for my parents. It's for everybody."

"Trans people wanted to share a story," James said, "and wanted to be heard and wanted to be acknowledged and wanted the rest of the United States and, dare I say it, the world to take notice that it's not about a very small percentage of the population. Trans people are everywhere."

The other takeaway from that press conference was from National Center for Transgender Equality Executive Director Mara Keisling. She said, "When people ask me what is the biggest issue for trans people I always say, 'It depends on which trans person you ask.'"

And there you have it. Transgender and nonbinary people are becoming more visible and are members of every community. They can help explain and humanize the numbers. And once you have heard one person's story, you have heard just one person's story. No one speaks for everyone. So, talk to several people, as we did for this guide. We found, and you will, too, that each person is different. But you will also find that we are all very much alike. Each of us has a desire and a right to be understood, to be accepted and to live our lives authentically.

—Joe Grimm

Selected Resources

BOOKS

Beemyn, Genny and Susan R. Rankin. *The Lives of Transgender People.* New York: Columbia University Press. 2011.

Beemyn, Genny. *Strategies for Supporting Trans and Gender-Nonconforming Youth.* AudioSolutionz. 2016. Audio CD.

Bilodeau, Brent. *Genderism: Transgender Students, Binary Systems and Higher Education.* Saarbrucken, Germany: VDM Verlag Dr. Müller. 2009.

Boedecker, Anne L. *The Transgender Guidebook: Keys to a Successful Transition.* Amazon Digital Services, LLC. 2011.

Bornstein, Kate and S. Bear Bergman. *Gender Outlaws: The Next Generation.* Seal Press reprint. 2010.

Bornstein, Kate. *My New Gender Workbook: A Step-by-Step Guide to Achieving World Peace Through Gender Anarchy and Sex Positivity (2nd edition)* London: Routledge. 2013.

Bornstein, Kate. *A Queer and Pleasant Danger: The True Story of a Nice Jewish Boy Who Joins the Church of Scientology, and Leaves Twelve Years Later to Become the Lovely Lady She is Today*. Boston: Beacon Press. 2013.

Boylan, Jennifer Finney. *She's Not There: A Life in Two Genders*. Broadway Books reprint. 2013.

Brill, Stephanie A. and Lisa Kinney. *The Transgender Teen*. Jersey City: Cleis Press. 2016.

Califia, Patrick. *Sex Changes: Transgender Politics (2nd edition)*. Jersey City: Cleis Press. 2003.

Erickson-Schroth, Laura, ed. *Trans Bodies, Trans Selves: A Resource for the Trans Community*. Oxford: Oxford University Press. 2014.

Erickson-Schroth, Laura and Laura A. Jacobs. *You're in the Wrong Bathroom!: And 20 Other Myths and Misconceptions About Transgender and Gender Nonconforming People*. Boston: Beacon Press. 2017.

Faludi, Susan. *In the Darkroom*. New York: Metropolitan Books. 2016.

Harrington, Lee. *Traversing Gender: Understanding Transgender Realities*. Anchorage: Mystic Productions Press. 2016.

Herman, Joanne. *Transgender Explained for Those Who are Not*. Bloomington: AuthorHouse. 2009.

Jennings, Jazz. *Being Jazz: My Life as a Transgender Teen*. New York: Crown Books for Young Readers. 2016.

Meyerowitz, Joanne. *How Sex Changed: A History of Transsexuality in the United States*. Cambridge: Harvard University Press. 2004.

Mock, Janet. *Redefining Realness: My Path to Womanhood, Identity, Love & So Much More*. New York: Atria Books reprint. 2014.

Nicolazzo, Z. *Trans* in College: Transgender Students' Strategies for Navigating Campus Life and the Institutional Politics of Inclusion*. Sterling: Stylus Publishing. 2016.

Nutt, Amy Ellis. *Becoming Nicole: The Transformation of an American Family*. New York: Random House Trade Paperbacks. 2016.

PFLAG. *Our Trans Loved Ones: Questions and Answers for Parents, Families, and Friends of People who are Transgender and Gender Expansive*. Washington, D.C. 2015. https://www.pflag.org/sites/default/files/Our%20Trans%20Loved%20Ones.pdf

Serano, Julia. *Whipping Girl: A Transsexual Woman on Sexism and the Scapegoating of Femininity (2nd edition)*. Berkeley: Seal Press. 2016.

Stryker, Susan. *Transgender History*. Berkeley: Seal Press. 2008.

Teich, Nicholas M. *Transgender 101: A simple Guide to a Complex Issue*. New York: Columbia University Press. 2012.

Valentine, David. *Imagining Transgender: An Ethnography of a Category*. Durham: Duke University Press. 2007.

JOURNALS, PUBLICATIONS AND STUDIES

The Advocate, http://www.advocate.com/

Grant, Jaime M., Lisa A. Mottet, Justin Tanis, Jack Harrison, Jody L. Herman and Mara Keisling. "Injustice at Every Turn: A Report of the National

Transgender Discrimination Survey." *Washington: National Center for Transgender Equality and National Gay and Lesbian Task Force. 2011.*

Gender Identity Project. *Transgender Basics.* New York: LGBT Community Center. 2009 update. Video.

GLQ: A Journal of Lesbian and Gay Studies, Duke University.

International Journal of Transgenderism (health and medicine), Routledge, 1998-present.

James, Sandy E., Jody L. Herman, Susan Rankin, Mara Keisling, Lisa Mottet and Ma'ayan Anaf. "The Report of the 2015 U.S. Transgender Survey." *Washington, D.C.: National Center for Transgender Equality.* 2016. http://www.ustranssurvey.org/

Jourian, T. J. "Evolving Nature of Sexual Orientation and Gender Identity." *New Directions for Student Services,* (152), 11-23. 2015.

Jourian, T. J. "Queering Constructs: Proposing a Dynamic Gender and Sexuality Model." *The Educational Forum* (Vol. 79, No. 4, pp. 459-474). Routledge. 2015.

Kosciw, J. G., E. A. Greytak, N. M. Giga, C. Villenas and D.J. Danischewski. "The 2015 National School Climate Survey: The Experiences of Lesbian, Gay, Bisexual, Transgender, and Queer Youth in Our Nation's Schools." *New York: GLSEN.* 2016.

Marine, S. B. and Z. Nicolazzo. Names That Matter: "Exploring the Tensions of Campus LGBTQ Centers and Trans* Inclusion." *Journal of Diversity in Higher Education,* 7(4), 265. 2014.

National Geographic. Special issue "Gender Revolution: The Shifting Landscape of Gender." Washington, D.C. January, 2017.

Nicolazzo, Z. and S. B. Marine. "It Will Change if People Keep Talking: Trans* Students in College and University Housing." *Journal of College and University Student Housing,* 42(1), 160-177. 2015.

Nicolazzo, Z. "It's a hard line to walk: Black Non-Binary Trans* Collegians' Perspectives on Passing, Realness, and Trans*-Normativity." *International Journal of Qualitative Studies in Education,* 1-16. 2016.

Nicolazzo, Z. D., E. N. Pitcher, K.A. Renn, and M. R. Woodford, M. R. (in press). "An Exploration of Trans* Kinship as a Strategy for Student Success." *Qualitative Studies in Education.*

The TransAdvocate http://transadvocate.com/

Transgender Studies Quarterly, Duke University Press, http://tsq.dukejournals.org/

ORGANIZATIONS

American Civil Liberties Union, LGBT rights, https://www.aclu.org/issues/lgbt-rights

Family Acceptance Project, https://familyproject.sfsu.edu/

GLAAD, http://www.glaad.org/

GLSEN.org: "Championing LGBTQ Issues in K-12 Education Since 1990"

Human Rights Campaign, http://www.hrc.org/

Intersex Society of North America, http://www.isna.org/

Lambda Legal, http://www.lambdalegal.org/

LGBT Resource Center, University of California-Riverside, http://www.out.ucr.edu/

National Center for Transgender Equality, http://www.transequality.org/

National Lesbian and Gay Journalists Association, http://www.nlgja.org/

Pew Research Center, http://www.pewresearch.org/

PFLAG, https://www.pflag.org/

Southern Poverty Law Center, LGBT rights, https://www.splcenter.org/issues/lgbt-rights

Stand with Trans, www.standwithtrans.org

Stonewall National Monument, https://www.nps.gov/ston/index.htm

Teaching Transgender Toolkit, http://www.teachingtransgender.org/authors/

Transgender Law Center, http://transgenderlawcenter.org/

Trans Murder Monitoring, research by Transgender Europe, http://transrespect.org/en/

Trans Student Educational Resources, http://www.transstudent.org/

TransWomen of Color Collective, http://www.twocc.us/

The Trevor Project, http://www.thetrevorproject.org/

Williams Institute, USLA College of Law, http://williamsinstitute.law.ucla.edu/

Our Story

The 100 Questions and Answers series springs from the idea that good journalism should increase cross-cultural competence and understanding. Most of our guides are created by Michigan State University journalism students.

We use journalistic interviews to surface the simple, everyday questions that people have about each other but might be afraid to ask. We use research and reporting to get the answers and then put them where people can find them, read them and learn about each other.

These cultural competence guides are meant to be conversation starters. We want people to use these guides to get some baseline understanding and to feel comfortable asking more questions. We put a resources section in every guide we make and we arrange community conversations. While the guides can answer questions in private, they are meant to spark discussions.

Making these has taught us that people are not that different from each other. People share more similarities than differences. We all want the same things for ourselves and for our families. We want to be accepted, respected and understood.

Please email your thoughts and suggestions to Series Editor Joe Grimm at joe.grimm@gmail.com, at the Michigan State University School of Journalism.

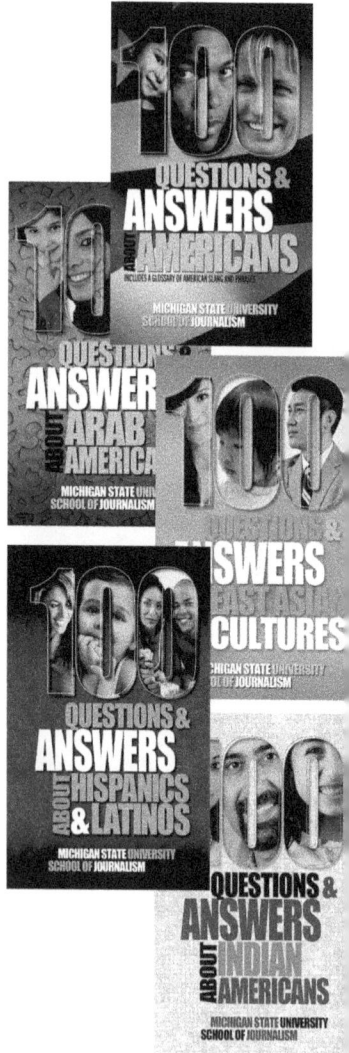

Related Books

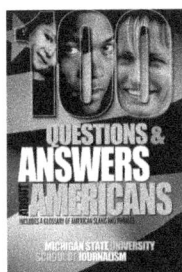

100 Questions and Answers About Americans
Michigan State University School of Journalism, 2013
This guide answers some of the first questions asked by newcomers to the United States. Questions represent dozens of nationalities coming from Africa, Asia, Australia, Europe and North and South America. Good for international students, guests and new immigrants.
http://news.jrn.msu.edu/culturalcompetence/

ISBN: 978-1-939880-20-8

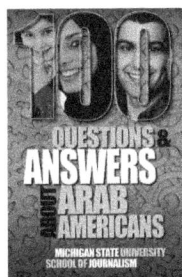

100 Questions and Answers About Arab Americans
Michigan State University School of Journalism, 2014
The terror attacks of Sept. 11, 2001, propelled these Americans into a difficult position where they are victimized twice. The guide addresses stereotypes, bias and misinformation. Key subjects are origins, religion, language and customs. A map shows places of national origin.
http://news.jrn.msu.edu/culturalcompetence/

ISBN: 978-1-939880-56-7

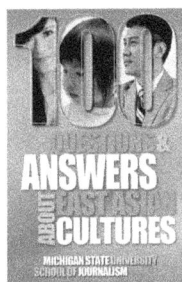

100 Questions and Answers About East Asian Cultures
Michigan State University School of Journalism, 2014
Large university enrollments from Asia prompted this guide as an aid for understanding cultural differences. The focus is on people from China, Japan, Korea and Taiwan and includes Mongolia, Hong Kong and Macau. The guide includes history, language, values, religion, foods and more.
http://news.jrn.msu.edu/culturalcompetence/

ISBN: 978-939880-50-5

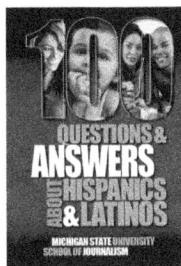

100 Questions and Answers About Hispanics & Latinos
Michigan State University School of Journalism, 2014
This group became the largest ethnic minority in the United States in 2014 and this guide answers many of the basic questions about it. Questions were suggested by Hispanics and Latinos. Includes maps and charts on origin and size of various Hispanic populations.
http://news.jrn.msu.edu/culturalcompetence/

ISBN: 978-1-939880-44-4

Print and ebooks available on Amazon.com and other retailers.

Related Books

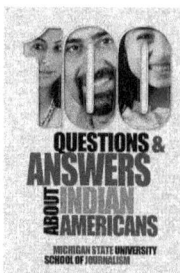

100 Questions and Answers About Indian Americans
Michigan State University School of Journalism, 2013
In answering questions about Indian Americans, this guide also addresses Pakistanis, Bangladeshis and others from South Asia. The guide covers religion, issues of history, colonization and national partitioning, offshoring and immigration, income, education, language and family.
http://news.jrn.msu.edu/culturalcompetence/

ISBN: 978-1-939880-00-0 m

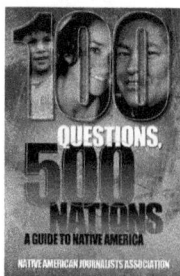

100 Questions, 500 Nations: A Guide to Native America
Michigan State University School of Journalism, 2014
This guide was created in partnership with the Native American Journalists Association. The guide covers tribal sovereignty, treaties and gaming, in addition to answers about population, religion, U.S. policies and politics. The guide includes the list of federally recognized tribes.
http://news.jrn.msu.edu/culturalcompetence/

ISBN: 978-1-939880-38-3

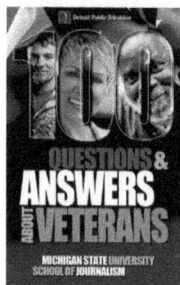

100 Questions and Answers About Veterans
Michigan State University School of Journalism, 2015
This guide treats the more than 20 million U.S. military veterans as a cultural group with distinctive training, experiences and jargon. Graphics depict attitudes, adjustment challenges, rank, income and demographics. Includes six video interviews by Detroit Public Television.
http://news.jrn.msu.edu/culturalcompetence/

ISBN: 978-1-942011-00-2

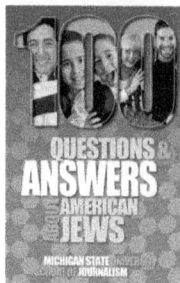

100 Questions and Answers About American Jews
Michigan State University School of Journalism 2016
We begin by asking and answering what it means to be Jewish in America. The answers to these wide-ranging, base-level questions will ground most people and set them up for meaningful conversations with Jewish acquaintants.
http://news.jrn.msu.edu/culturalcompetence/

ISBN: 978-1-942011-22-4

Print and ebooks available on Amazon.com and other retailers.

Related Books

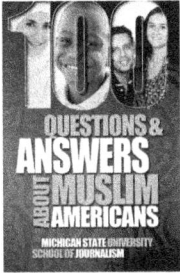

100 Questions and Answers About Muslim Americans
Michigan State University School of Journalism, 2014
This guide was done at a time of rising intolerance in
the United States toward Muslims. The guide describes
the presence of this religious group around the world
and inside the United States. It includes audio on
how to pronounce some basic Muslim words.
http://news.jrn.msu.edu/culturalcompetence/

ISBN: 978-1-939880-79-6

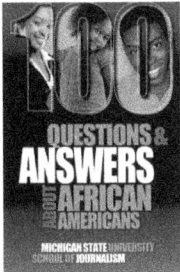

100 Questions and Answers About African Americans
Michigan State University School of Journalism, 2016
Learn about the racial issues that W.E.B. DuBois said in
1900 would be the big challenge for the 20th century.
This guide explores Black and African American identity,
history, language, contributions and more. Learn more
about current issues in American cities and campuses.
http://news.jrn.msu.edu/culturalcompetence/

ISBN: 978-1-942011-19-4

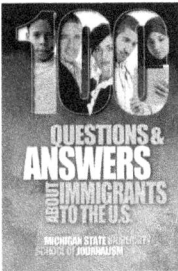

100 Questions and Answers About Immigrants to the U.S.
Michigan State University School of Journalism 2016
This simple, introductory guide answers 100 of the
basic questions people ask about U.S. immigrants
and immigration in everyday conversation. It
has answers about identity, language, religion,
culture, customs, social norms, economics,
politics, education, work, families and food.

ISBN: 978-1-934879-63-4

THE NEW BULLYING

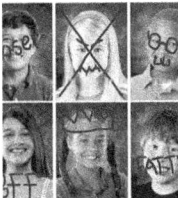

The New Bullying
Bullying has changed considerably. This book is
intended to document that change. Among the changes
that were examined are the rise of cyberbullying,
social exclusion as a form of bullying, new laws
about school bullying, computer crimes and threats
and a growing willingness on the part of the public
to talk about bullying and its perceived connection
to suicide and violence, especially in schools.

HOW SOCIAL MEDIA, SOCIAL EXCLUSION, LAWS AND
SUICIDE CHANGED BULLYING

ISBN: 978-1-934879-63-4

Print and ebooks available on Amazon.com and other retailers.

www.ingramcontent.com/pod-product-compliance
Lightning Source LLC
Chambersburg PA
CBHW021625270326
41931CB00008B/869